This journal belongs to

____